AN ALZHEIMER'S LOVE STORY

A Musical Preparation/Proposal

By: Michael A. Horvich

ISBN

9 781304 336507

May 2019
Michael A. Horvich, Creativity Ltd
807 Davis Street Suite 415
Evanston, Illinois 60201
Follow Michael at: http://www.horvich.com

AN ALZHEIMER'S LOVE STORY

A Musical Preparation/Proposal

By: Michael A. Horvich

ALZHEIMER'S

A MUSICAL LOVE STORY

Love, Life, & Liberation

By Michael A. Horvich & Gregory L. Maire

WORKING TITLES

GREGORY:

An Alzheimer's LOVE STORY

Love, Life, & Liberation

By Michael A. Horvich & Gregory L. Maire

<u>DEDICATION</u>

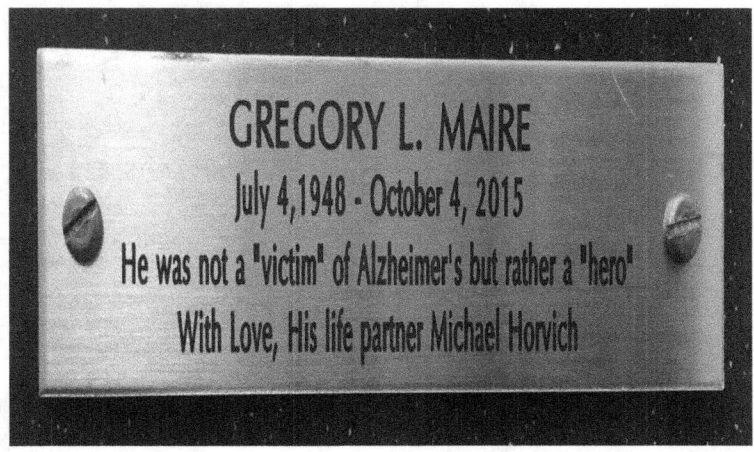

Memorial plaque at Liberman Memory Care Facility:

He was not a "**VICTIM**" OF ALZHEIMER'S but rather a "**HERO**"

Gregory did not "**SUFFER**" with Alzheimer's,
rather he "**LIVED**" as well as possible with the disease.

This musical documentation is dedicated to Gregory Lee Maire,

my husband of 41 years, 1976-2015,

whose death taught me what grieving was really all about!

✳✳✳

THANK YOU

To Gregory and all those family and friends who have encouraged me over the years to be more of who I am.

To Gigi, my kitty and those who have moved on: Broadway, Hoover, Mariah, and Emma.

To Mark and Colleen Maire, my nephew and niece-in-law, to whom I trust my life … and fact I do and have made them my power of attorney over health care and trustees and executors of my estate!

To the Ragdale Foundation for acceptance to their juried, competitive application, two week residency program which gave me encouragement, time, & space to write & for helping to give me emotional permission to call myself "An Artist". 2010

To Chicago Children's Museum on Navy Pier, for lovingly inviting "Michael's Museum: A Curious Collection of Tiny Treasures" to become a permanent exhibit at the museum. 2011.

To Patricia Anderson, good friend, and fellow writer, for being a good friend to Gregory as well and for taking the photo of Gregory and me crying together which I have used often in my publications.

To www.medium.com and Prism & Pen for giving the LGBTQ Community a place to share their stories and a platform for me to share mine. And thanks to my primary editors James Finn (Essays) and Esther Jones (Poetry).

❋❋❋

OPENING QUOTES

LOVE: The greatest thing you'll ever learn is just to love and be loved in return. *From the song Nature Boy by Eden Ahbez. 1947. Popularized in the movie and Broadway musical: Moulin Rouge.*

ALIVENESS: The source of continuing aliveness is to find your passion and to pursue it with whole heart and single mind. *Modern Maturity Magazine. Gail Sheehy. July 1995.*

CELEBRATION: To live is to change, to acquire the words of a story, and that is the only celebration we mortals really know. *The Poisonwood Bible. Barbara Kingsolver. 2002. P 385.*

COLLECTING: All collections try to elude time. To stop time, to control time. Collecting is the closest thing to immortality—which is, of course, the irony of it because the collector is physical, which is to say temporal. The collector is a childlike figure, a prisoner of the eternal present. *Rephrased: The Secret of Lost Things. Sheridan Hay. P 112.*

LIFE: I now know why I like musicals and opera. Life is meant to be sung! *M. Horvich 2008*

DYING: It always ends Happily Ever After! *M. Horvich 2004*

DEATH: Spirits know where to fly when it's time, there's no reason to mourn! *Author Unknown*

GRIEF: No one ever told me that grief felt so like fear. C.S. Lewis from School for the Blind By: Dennis McFarland. 1995.

✳✳✳

DEAR READER

Namasté

I honor the place in you in which
the entire universe dwells.
I honor the place in you which is of love,
of truth, of light and of peace.
When you are in that place in you and
I am in that place in me, we are one.

✳✳✳

TABLE OF CONTENTS

AN ALZHEIMER'S LOVE STORY

A Musical Preparation/Proposal

By: Michael A. Horvich

ALZHEIMER'S

A MUSICAL LOVE STORY

Love, Life, & Liberation

By Michael A. Horvich & Gregory L. Maire

WORKING TITLES

GREGORY:

An Alzheimer's LOVE STORY

Love, Life, & Liberation

By Michael A. Horvich & Gregory L. Maire

BRIEF PITCH

ALZHEIMER'S
A MUSICAL LOVE STORY
Love, Life, & Liberation
By Michael A. Horvich & Gregory L. Maire

WORKING TITLES

GREGORY:
An Alzheimer's LOVE STORY
Love, Life, & Liberation
By Michael A. Horvich & Gregory L. Maire

BRIEF PITCH

ALZHEIMER'S: The Musical Love Story
or
GREORY: An Alzheimer's Musical Love Story

By Michael A. Horvich and Gregory Maire

One story weaving together three tapestries: A beautiful love relationship, living well with Alzheimer's Disease, and tracing Gay Liberation Events from the early 1960's through today.

Raw and honest but compassionate and up-lifting. Gives hope to living a life well when confronted by a disease which is progressively hopeless.

SYNOPSIS:

PROLOGUE: The musical opens with the cast on stage before the overture, warming up, conversing with each other, and possibly acknowledging people they see in the audience. Michael begins to share, as everyone on stage leaves, the background of the story the audience is about to witness.

OVERTURE:

ACT ONE: Gregory and Michael meet during the 70's when the Equal Rights Amendment was once again stirring people to action. Men are beginning to question their feminine side and women are again beginning to resent being second class citizens. LGBTQ life was just beginning to be more visible and slightly more acceptable. Gregory was married to a woman and Michael was in a long-term relationship with a man. Both of their lives were beginning to change including leaving their current spouses behind for each other.

ACT TWO: Gregory and Michael make a commitment to each other and as societal acceptance of homosexuality grows, so in parallel does their love grow. They experience a new freedom to be who they are and to love whom they choose. Gay bath house sex is more available, STDs are on the rise, being able to dance and socialize in public is on the increase. The LGBTQ Community continues working on civil freedoms and taking care of their own, HIV/AIDS shows up as the "Gay Cancer" and eventually is realized to be everyone's concern, Civil Unions are taking place in more and more states, eventually Same Sex Marriage is the rule of law.

ACT THREE: In the 29th year of their 41 year relationship, Alzheimer's Disease moves in as the uninvited third partner to Ménage à trois. Gregory and Michael recommit to each other and declare that they love each other "More Than Ever." As Gregory's cognitive abilities diminish, Michael is more creative with how to support him. Normalcy in their life becomes more difficult to find but they prevail.

ACT FOUR: Eventually Gregory moves to a Memory Care Facility and Michael visits every day. After Gregory's living with Alzheimer's Disease for twelve years, and Michael walking the Alzheimer's Path with him, Gregory dies.

EPILOGUE: Michael laments his death but also celebrates Gregory's life as Michael expounds on some of his Buddhist learnings.

NOTES:

As this musical is developed, the lyrics and music will bring the story to life more than just the scene synopses are able to do.

Dances includes: Ballet, Jazz, Rock, Tap, Modern, Swing, Ballroom.

Musical numbers include as many genres as possible

Highlights:
> Growth of Love Relationship
> Depth of Relationship
> Relationship roles Change or Develop According to Strengths
> Dementia/Alzheimer's Disease Diagnosis and discussion
> Lying Down and Dying or Hunkering Down and Living
> Living Well After Diagnosis with Alzheimer's
> Alzheimer's Doesn't Have to Be A Death Sentence
> Falling In Love Again Each and Every Day
> Joy/Sorrow
> Life/Death/Grief

Events:
> Stonewall
> First Gay Pride Parade
> Gay Bath House Sex
> Disco/Drag Queen Performance
> HIV/AIDS
> Gay March on Washington
> Vermont Civil Union/Same Sex Marriage

❋❋❋

INTRODUCTION

ALZHEIMER'S

A MUSICAL

LOVE STORY

Love, Life, & Liberation

By Michael A. Horvich & Gregory L. Maire

WORKING TITLES

GREGORY:

An Alzheimer's

LOVE STORY

Love, Life, & Liberation

By Michael A. Horvich & Gregory L. Maire

INTRODUCTION

(Working titles)

"GREGORY: A Musical Love Story: Love Life and Liberation"

or

"ALZHEIMER'S: A Musical Love Story Love Life and Liberation"

By Michael A. Horvich

m@horvich.com
www.horvich.com
847-738-1776

One story weaving together three tapestries: A beautiful love relationship, living well with Alzheimer's Disease, and tracing Gay Liberation Events from the early 1960's through today.

Raw and honest but compassionate and up-lifting. Gives hope to living life well when confronted by a disease which is uncurable and progressively hopeless.

A MUSICAL IN FOUR ACTS

Prologue – Today—2020

Act One: The Beginning—1960's

Act Two: The Middle 1980's—2000

Intermission

Act Three: The Beginning of the End—2003/2014

Act Four: Great Love Means Great Grief—2014/15

CHARACTERS

GREGORY, co-protagonist diagnosed with Alzheimer's.
Tall, thin, fair, blondish hair, good looking, intelligent, thoughtful, calm, and soft spoken. Starts at age 30, with

Dementia diagnosis at 55, and ages to 68. Played by two actors (younger & older.)

MICHAEL, co-protagonist, life partner to Gregory. Short, heavy, dark, black hair, good looking, enthusiastic and not afraid to speak, hyper, sometimes too loud. Starts out at 33 years old and currently 71. Played by two actors (younger & older.)

MGC = MALE GREEK CHORUS (6) – All ages, some buff, some out of shape
Variously: Monday Night Men's Gathering Group, Gay Family, Friends, Crowds

FGC = FEMALE GREEK CHORUS (6) – All ages, some svelte, some "big girls"
Variously: Crowd, Family, Friends

TREATMENT/SYNOPSIS

PROLOGUE: The musical opens with the cast on empty stage before the overture, warming up, conversing with each other, and possibly acknowledging people they see in the audience. Purpose is to remove, temporarily, the "Fourth Wall." Everyone leaves stage in darkness as spot light picks up Michael sitting in a winged back chair. He begins to share the background of the story which the audience is about to witness, a true representation of the characters' experiences with their developing love for each other, the changing acceptance of Gay Life, and the joys and sorrows of living well with Dementia/Alzheimer's Disease.

OVERTURE: Dynamic music moving from beautiful and melodic to chaotic as it progresses.

ACT ONE: Gregory and Michael meet during the 70's when the Equal Rights Amendment was once again stirring people to action thinking about the intersecting roles of men and women. Men are beginning to question their feminine side and women are again resenting being second class citizens. LGBTQ life was just beginning to be more visible and slightly more acceptable. Often hate crimes occur with Gays as the victims. Gregory is married to a woman and Michael is in a long-term relationship with a man. Both of Michael and Gregory's lives are beginning to change including leaving their current **spouses behind for each other.**

ACT TWO: Gregory and Michael make a commitment to each other and as societal acceptance of homosexuality grows, so in parallel does their love grow. They experience a new freedom to be who they are and live a life in which "love is love." Gay bars, meeting places, and bath house sex is more available, STDs are on the rise. **The LGBTQ Community continues** working on civil freedoms and taking care of their own, HIV/AIDS shows up as the "Gay Cancer" and eventually is realized to be everyone's concern, Civil Unions are taking place in more and more states, eventually Same Sex Marriage is the rule of law. Gay life slowly is becoming more visible on TV, in movies, and on the streets with Gays in positive roles.

ACT THREE: In the 29th year of their 41 year relationship, Alzheimer's Disease moves in as the uninvited third partner to a Ménage à trois_. Gregory and Michael recommit to each other and declare that they love each other "More Than Ever."** As Gregory's cognitive abilities diminish, Michael is more creative with how to support him. **Respect continues to be the measure of their relationship.** Normalcy in their life becomes more difficult to maintain but they prevail.

ACT FOUR: Eventually Gregory moves to a Memory Care Facility and Michael visits every day. Same-sex marriage becomes law but at this point in their life, Michael and Gregory decide it is not in their best interests to wed. After Gregory's living with Alzheimer's Disease for twelve years, and Michael walking the Alzheimer's Path with him, Gregory dies peacefully.

EPILOGUE: Michael laments Gregory's death but also celebrates Gregory's life as Michael expounds on some of his Buddhist learnings primarily the Heart Sutra. (An alternative ending is revisiting the major milestones in Gay Liberation with dynamic music and colorful lights.)

DETAILS

HIGHLIGHTS:

Great Differences Provide Great Strengths
Growth and Depth of Love Relationship
Relationship roles Change or Develop According to Strengths
Dementia/Alzheimer's Disease Diagnosis and Discussion
Living Well After Diagnosis with Alzheimer's
Alzheimer's Doesn't Have to Be A Death Sentence
Falling In Love Again Each and Every Day
Progression of Dementia and Loss of Cognitive Abilities
Dependence/Independence/Joy/Sorrow/Life/Death/Grief

EVENTS:

Stonewall
First Gay Pride Parade
Gay Bath House Sex
Disco/Drag Queen Performance
Howard Brown Health Clinic
HIV/AIDS
Gay March on Washington
Vermont Civil Union/Same Sex Marriage

MUSIC:

Jazz, Ballad, Ballet, Disco, Torch Song, Classical, Hip Hop, Western, Folk, Blues

DANCE:

Ballet, Tap, Ballroom, Jazz, Modern, Tango, Rhumba, Samba, Mambo

SCENE LIST

PROLOGUE 2019

OVERTURE

ACT 1 – BEGINNING: 1970's
1.1   Stonewall Riots (1959) / Gay Life (1960s)
1.2   Monday Night Gathering: Gregory and Michael Meet (1974)
1.3   Love Grows / First Kiss (1976)

✳✳✳

THE MUSICAL SYNOPSIS

ALZHEIMER'S
A MUSICAL LOVE STORY
Love, Life, & Liberation
By Michael A. Horvich & Gregory L. Maire

WORKING TITLES

GREGORY:
An Alzheimer's LOVE STORY
Love, Life, & Liberation
By Michael A. Horvich & Gregory L. Maire

THE MUSICAL SYNOPSIS: A MUSICAL IN FOUR ACTS

Prologue – Today—2019

Act One: The Beginning—1960's

Act Two: The Middle 1980's—2000

Intermission

Act Three: The Beginning of the End—2003—2014

Act Four: Great Love Means Great Grief—2014/15

CHARACTER LIST

GREGORY, the co-protagonist diagnosed with Alzheimer's. Tall, thin, fair, blondish hair, good looking, intelligent, thoughtful, calm, and soft spoken. Starts out at 30 years old and ages to 68. May be 2 actors.

MICHAEL, the co-protagonist, life partner to Gregory. Short, heavy, dark, black hair, good looking, enthusiastic and not afraid to speak, hyper, sometimes too loud. Starts out at 33 years old and ends up at 71. May be 2 actors.

MGC = MALE GREEK CHORUS (6) – All ages, some buff, some out of shape

Variously: Monday Night Men's Gathering Group, Gay Family, Friends, Crowds

FGC = FEMALE GREEK CHORUS (6) – All ages, some svelte, some "big girls"

Variously: Crowd, Jan, Cheryl, Patricia

SCENE LIST

PROLOGUE 2019

OVERTURE

ACT 1 – BEGINNING: 1970's

1.1   Stonewall Riots (1959) / Gay Life (1960s)

1.2   Monday Night Gathering: Gregory and Michael Meet (1974)

1.3   Love Grows / First Kiss (1976)

1.4   First Ever Gay Pride Parade (1970) "Walk Across"

1.5   Man's Country Bath House (1970's)

ACT 2 – MIDDLE: 1980's, 1990's, 2000's

2.1   DISCO (1980's)

2.2   A Visit to Howard Brown Clinic (1980's)

2.3   HIV/AIDS (1980's)

2.4   I Love You (1990's)

2.5   Second Gay March on Washington (1993)

2.6   Walk Across: Gay Pride Parade (2000's)

2.7   Vermont Civil Union (2000)

ACT 3 – BEGINNING OF THE END: 2003 - 2014

3.1   The Diagnosis (2003)

3.2   Walk Across: More Than Ever (2005)

3.3   Living with Alzheimer's (2007

3.4   Living with More Alzheimer's (2011)

3.5   Walk Across: Gregory's Decline (2013)

3.6   How Can I Go On? (2014)

ACT 4 – THE END: 2014/15

4.1   A Song Without Words (2014)

Besides Old Michael announcing and explaining some of the scenes, a placard could be lowered from the ceiling or travel across the stage, perhaps pushed by Old Michael as he enters with the name of the scene, a date, and/or a newspaper headline.

THE MUSICAL

ALZHEIMER'S
A MUSICAL
LOVE STORY
Love, Life, & Liberation
By Michael A. Horvich & Gregory L. Maire

WORKING TITLES

GREGORY:
An Alzheimer's
LOVE STORY
Love, Life, & Liberation
By Michael A. Horvich & Gregory L. Maire

PROLOGUE

ALZHEIMER'S

A MUSICAL LOVE STORY

Love, Life, & Liberation

By Michael A. Horvich & Gregory L. Maire

WORKING TITLES

GREGORY:

An Alzheimer's LOVE STORY

Love, Life, & Liberation

By Michael A. Horvich & Gregory L. Maire

PROLOGUE – 2015

As audience fills the house, the curtain is up. Stage is empty with back brick wall showing. About ten minutes before the show, the actors begin entering the stage and begin warming up. Stretching. Voice exercises. Etc. They greet each other, notice the audience, wave at someone, whatever. Somewhat spontaneous.

Old Michael, is also on stage warming up with the others.

Michael sits in a winged-back chair, center stage as the house light dim and a spot comes up on him. Others exit. (Projection of Michael and Gregory on screen lowered on back wall "ALZHEIMER'S: A Love Story.") The time is today and Michael is 73 years old.

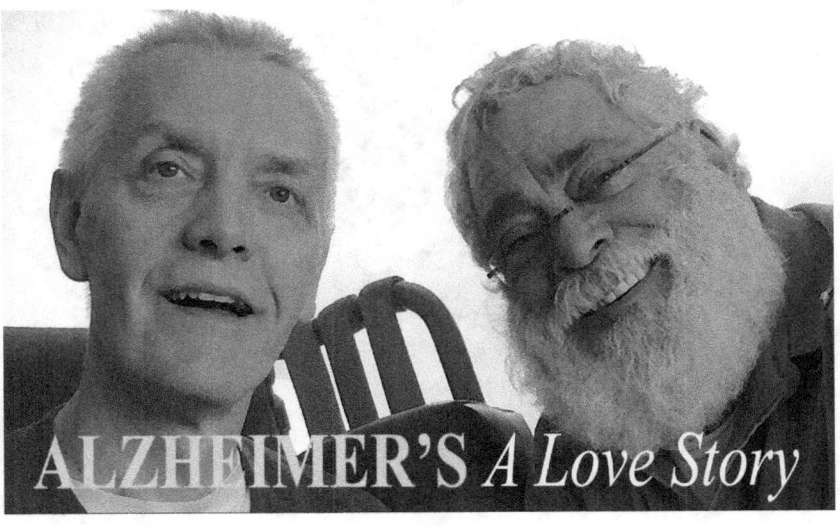

NARRATOR (OLD MICHAEL) : Sets the stage for the musical

Hi. Welcome. Pleased you could make it this evening. The story I am about to tell you is absolutely true. Every detail … well most details anyway ... as many as I can remember accurately!

Some I may have forgotten and others may be too painful to remember. Anyway, **I know** because I am not only **telling** you the story, but I **lived** it. **We** lived it. Gregory, my life partner, my husband, of over **41 years** and I **lived** it. (*Deep breath and sigh and hesitates.*)

If I begin to cry … no, I am not afraid to cry in front of you, … but it is hell trying to talk and cry at the same time. So, if I do get choked up, I'll stop, take a few deep breaths, and be back with you before you even notice that I have been gone.

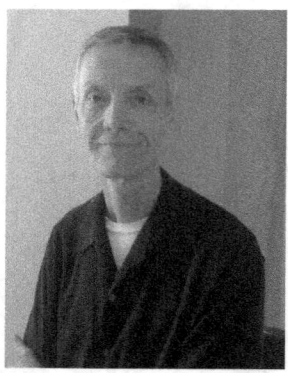

Picture of Gregory comes up on screen. Glancing over his left shoulder looking at it, Michael continues ...

That photograph. That's a picture that I took of Gregory many years ago and is what I call my "stock photo" of Gregory during his best times.

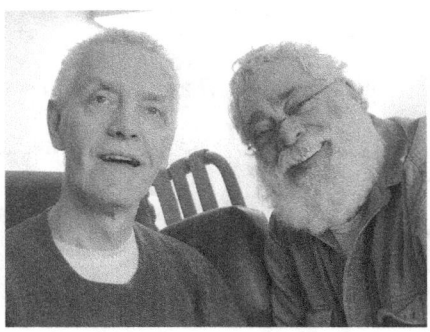

(Photo changes) This is my "stock photo" of the more difficult, yet still happy times. (Projection of Michael with Gregory in wheel chair.)

Slowly, diagnosed with Dementia/Alzheimer' at 55 years old, over twelve years Gregory lost his ability to talk, to feed himself, to be mobile. Most of his abilities slowly left us. I never referred to the diagnosis as his, I always called it **our** diagnosis of Dementia, most likely Alzheimer'

Now I **don't** want you to feel sad for us … Gregory lived well during the time he had left and I was able to support and love him, as he loved me. As we used to say, "I love you more than ever!"

It wasn't an easy path to walk, but we prevailed, even though at times we didn't anticipate the roller coaster turns our life would take!

The diagnosis of Alzheimer's, does not have to be a death sentence … and be certain that Gregory did not "suffer" with Alzheimer's, rather with my help, he lived as well as possible. He was **NOT** a **VICTIM** of Alzheimer's … he was a **HERO**!

Lately as I tell my story, I have been able to say (*voice cracking*) that neither Gregory or I were **VICTIMS**, we were **BOTH** heroes.

Blackout

OVERTURE

ALZHEIMER'S

A MUSICAL LOVE STORY

Love, Life, & Liberation

By Michael A. Horvich & Gregory L. Maire

WORKING TITLES

GREGORY:

An Alzheimer's LOVE STORY

Love, Life, & Liberation

By Michael A. Horvich & Gregory L. Maire

OVERTURE

MUSIC

The overture begins slowly and gets louder and louder and more and more chaotic. The music is Fellini/circus like.

ACT ONE

ALZHEIMER'S

A MUSICAL LOVE STORY

Love, Life, & Liberation

By Michael A. Horvich & Gregory L. Maire

WORKING TITLES

GREGORY:

An Alzheimer's LOVE STORY

Love, Life, & Liberation

By Michael A. Horvich & Gregory L. Maire

ACT ONE SCENE ONE

Stonewall Riots / Gay Nightlife
(1959—1960)

Slide show of Gay Life in the 50's and 60's followed by slides showing the Stonewall Riots shown on screen back stage.

OLD MICHAEL NARRATOR:

During the 50' and 60's, Gay Life was nothing like it is today. Most gays were closeted, living in secret, even married with children because it was what society expected. There were no gay role models in the movies, on TV, or in the literature of the day. Only in Illinois was it <u>not</u> a criminal act to engage in what they called Homosexual acts, that was before the term Gay was coined. It was called "The Love That Dare Not Speak Its Name."

On a hot summer night in 1969, police raided the Stonewall Inn, a bar located in New York City's Greenwich Village that served as a haven for the city's gay, lesbian, and transgender community.

At the time, homosexual acts remained illegal in every state except Illinois, and bars and restaurants could get shut down for having gay employees or serving gay patrons. Most gay bars and clubs in New York at the time (including the Stonewall) were operated by the Mafia, who paid corruptible police officers to look the other way and blackmailed wealthy gay patrons by threatening to "out" them.

Police raids on gay bars were common, but on that particular night, members of the city's LGBT community decided to fight back—sparking an uprising that would launch a new era of resistance and revolution.

During 60's, Gay night life was pretty much hidden from view. *(Action goes on as the narrator describes)* Imagine walking down a dark alley to a door above which hangs no sign or any indication as to what is behind the door. Knock several times, a small hatch opens and if you look "OK" to the person behind the door he lets you in. A roughly constructed bar runs along one side of the room, bathrooms are towards the back, next to the door stands a juke box playing dance music. There are one hundred or more gay men and women in the bar; visiting, drinking, and dancing. The bar is about to be raided. Watch what happens. Welcome to "Bob's Bistro" on Wells Street in Chicago.

MUSIC

Music of the 50's and 60's playing, the quality of stereo on a jukebox.

SETTING

People are visiting, cruising, drinking, and dancing. The scene lasts long enough to demonstrate the type of dancing people did during that time. Suddenly and unexpectedly, the door person announces in a loud voice, "RAID!" The door is bashed open and by the time the police enter the bar, it is obvious that all of the gay men, who have been dancing with other men, grab a woman dancing partner and vice versa for the women.

POLICE MAN IN CHARGE:

Alright take out your ID. If you are underage, you are in trouble. If we suspect you are using drugs, you are in trouble. If we don't like your looks, you are in trouble. You will be finger printed and your name will appear in the newspaper. *Chaos ensues, some people try to escape, some run to the bathrooms, some are cuffed, some are dragged out by the collar to the waiting vans.*

ACT ONE SCENE TWO

Monday Night Meeting

Gregory and Michael Meet

(1970's)

OLD MICHAEL NARRATOR:

During the 70's slowly progress was made in attitudes towards and accepting of people who were Gay. They were able to live a little more openly, a little more freely. In general, many men, gay and straight, began to take a closer look at who they were in relation to women. It slowly was becoming OK for men to acknowledge their feminine side, to help with household chores, to help take care of the children. The roles of men and women at home and in the workplace were slowly changing.

Groups of men met in what were called sensitivity groups, consisting of men who were old, young, married, divorced, single, gay, and straight formed groups who met weekly to discuss issues, emotions, changes, etc. The joining together of men from various interests and beliefs proved a great place for each of them to grow and be more accepting of others and of themselves. It turns out that Gregory and Michael met at one such sensitivity group meeting. Let's watch.

SETTING:

A non-descript living room with (MGC – Male Greek Chorus) and Michael, all members of the Monday Night Group of The Men's Gathering, a 1970's awareness group. Gay, straight, black, white, Latino, Asian, old young, single, married, divorced. All those present are visiting, sipping a drink or glass of wine, eating snacks.

Gregory walks into the room, all freeze as Michael notices him, Michael stands, room lights dim with spots picking up Michael and Gregory in spots at opposite sides of the room, romantically lit. Michael is 33 years old and Gregory is 30 years old.

MUSICAL NUMBER:

Gregory and Michael sing. Deals with love at first sight, lust, but also deeper feeling that this match is an important one. Reminiscent of the scene in West Side Story *at the dance.*

Lighting and action return to normal and group meeting begins.

DIALOGUE TBD (To Be Developed)

Conversation of the group at the meeting deals with the kind of issues with which they deal: Monogamy vs fidelity to spouses, accepting their feminine side, self-confidence, gay issues vs straight issues, etc

POSSIBLE MUSICAL NUMBER 2:

Deals with growing pride in self. Throwing off what other's think, cultural norms, familial ought's and should's. Similar to "I Am What I Am" from La Cage Aux Folles.

ACT ONE SCENE THREE
Their Love Grows

(1970)

OLD MICHAEL NARRATOR: DIALOGUE: (TBD)

Talks about being Gay in the 70's and the continued risks in a largely unaccepting society.

SETTING

A series of vignettes in front of the curtain in which Michael and Gregory get to know each other and fall in love. However, their interactions not being too overt because of the times. Moving across stage (one of several future "walk arounds.") Possibly a turntable or moving walk (or possibly two.)

Having dinner at home, attending a movie, having a drink at a bar, watching TV, exchanging back rubs, sharing a book, grocery shopping, talking, on the beach, exchanging a kiss now and then, etc.

MUSIC

Passage of time, falling in love while still not publicly accepted. Learning to accept oneself even though not accepted by family, society, etc. How do you measure love and life as it grows in a year or in a lifetime? Or could be instrumental showing passage of time. Or Sung by MGC and FGC who also interact with M&G and cross stage periodically in opposite directions; people at the theater, grocery store, at beach, in bar, etc.

SETTING

All items precede Michael and Gregory off stage right. Michael and Gregory end up stage left, hand in hand for the first time as stage lights dim and alley projection and back-alley door prop comes on. Just before they arrive at a door, a shout of "FAGGOT" comes angrily from off stage, Gregory and Michael back into doorway to be unseen. A young kid runs, scared, looking back over his shoulder, across from stage left and off at stage right. (Possibly being chased by two rough teens with baseball bats.)

Michael and Gregory step back into the light of the street facing each other, a little nervous but calming each other, left hand in left hand and right hand in right hand.

MUSIC

They sing about having to hide their love from others, from society and the difficulty of having to damper the feelings of such a strong love and "to kiss in the shadows." Wanting to kiss when you want to kiss, holding hands, touching, caressing without regard for where you are or who is around, but not being able to do so for fear of getting beaten up, fired from your job, tossed out by family.

ACT ONE SCENE FOUR
Walk Across: First Gay Pride Parade (1970)

SETTING

In contrast to the peppy music, straggly parade, widely separated, obviously only a few participants, a number of police men along route, smaller group of observers behind blockades, some supportive,

others indifferent, and possibly hostile. Marchers carrying signs,
American flags upside down, drag queens, others dressed gay of the
day. Not much energy, not much enthusiasm, more a protest than a
celebratory parade. (Marchers will enter stage right, cross, exit stage
left, drop prop, cross behind curtain, pick up new prop, enter again.)
Parade ends with several of the observers yelling anti-gay remarks
and throwing garbage. Police enter become more active. Slow black
out.

DIALOGUE: (TBD) OLD MICHAEL NARRATOR

Talks about the Stonewall Riots and the emerging beginnings of "Gay
Pride" and the Rainbow Flag. The first Gay Pride Parade was an
important event although one with fear, some violence, and great risk.

MUSIC

In front of curtain, peppy marching type music.

ACT ONE SCENE FIVE
Man's Country Bath House

(1970's)

SETTING

Lights come up on Michael and Gregory, wearing only towels,
standing in a darkish hallway with overhead warehouse type hanging

lights and a series of room doors numbered 1 – 2 – 3 etc. A logo type sign painted on the wall indicates "Bath House."

On the other side of the hallway is one larger door, opening into another room (the orgy room) which is basically without any light (just enough to barely see people moving around.)

Periodically someone walks down the hallway and out, sometimes down the hallway and into the "other room,' naked with a towel around their waist. A couple enters one of the rooms.

DIALOGUE: (TBD) OLD MICHAEL NARRATOR

Talks about sexuality of the time. Very few places Gay men could meet and Bath Houses where they could "hook up" with other men to meet, make friends, and/or for sexual adventures.

Welcome to Man's Country on Clark Street.

MUSIC

Background music 70's disco dance type.

DIALOGUE MICHAEL & GREGORY: (TBD)

In the locker room of the bath house Michael talks to Gregory (who is the thoughtful one and new to the gay life) about the need to experience a new situation before one can be thoughtful and analyze one's feeling about the experience and/or make any decisions about how they want to behave in these situations.

Music swells, as Gregory goes through to orgy room. Michael stays in place, watches a stranger come down the hall and go into the orgy room. Michael follows.

During musical interlude as all lights slowly fade to black. "Sex" moans and groans, etc. Lighting in Orgy Room could be just enough to see shadows engaged in "dance oriented" sex. Lights slowly go back dim and then to original as music fades. Voices of two men, apparently having "hooked up," are heard coming from the orgy room. They are still in the dark as they exit, you can see their shape but nothing more. One is tall and slender; one is short and heavier. The two men pause talking about "What a great experience!" thanking each other, and as they continue into the light, you realize that the two men are Gregory and Michael. They react with surprise and laughter!

Michael and Gregory, still at the bath house in their towels, walk over to a table in the "Café" having purchased a soda and chips. Behind them is the bath house service counter with the server. Men, some single and some in couples, all in towels, come in and out, walking by, etc.

DIALOGUE MICHAEL & GREGORY: (TBD)

They talk about the experience, Gregory processing his feelings, and the emotional/social benefits of being a same sex couple. They decide to go home and fuck.

ACT II

ALZHEIMER'S

A MUSICAL

LOVE STORY

Love, Life, & Liberation

By Michael A. Horvich & Gregory L. Maire

WORKING TITLES

GREGORY:

An Alzheimer's

LOVE STORY

Love, Life, & Liberation

By Michael A. Horvich & Gregory L. Maire

ACT TWO SCENE ONE
DISCO
(1980's)

OLD MICHAEL NARRATOR

Let's jump ahead ten years. Life for the Gay Community has gotten a little better. They can be more visible, there are TV programs which deal with Gay life, there are places to go to meet people, to have a drink, to dance the night away. Some people, some of the time, in some parts of their life can be "out." Join us at "The Bistro," at Dearborn and Hubbard Streets, Chicago's first New York-style discotheque with a predominately Gay if not "hip" clientele. There is a sign out front and a clean, exciting inside! Gregory and Michael are out partying with friends.

SETTING

Lights come up on a mirror balled, flashing lights dance floor center stage. Disco music is blaring. There is a bar and stools center and upper stage right. People are sitting and milling about, drinking, smoking. People are on the dance floor dancing. Michael and Gregory (in follow spot so they are noticed but not so bright as to distract from disco mood) enter downstage right, greet several friends, and order a drink from the bartender. A popular song comes up and everyone excitedly run to the dance floor. The music lasts long enough to demonstrate "disco dancing:" hot, sweaty, sexual, many men without shirts.

MUSIC

Disco music. Could be a compilation of parts of many popular disco pieces of the 80's.

SETTING

Some kind of triumphant music announces the beginning of the next song, people who have been on the dance floor back off as spot lights pick up a platform descending from the ceiling. All eyes are on the platform on which is an "over the top" drag queen

MUSIC

Lip syncing a popular 80's ABBA type piece or something like "It's Raining Men."

After her piece, as the platform slowly ascends, when the next piece of music begins, people hoot, and yell, and run to the dance floor dancing dances of the era, period of wonderful dancing, light show, mirror ball, loud music, to wildly disappear into the music. The piece could include a few bars from each of the popular songs of the day. Extended, Interesting choreography piece ends this scene.

✳✳✳

ACT TWO SCENE TWO
A Visit to Howard Brown Clinic
(1980's)

OLD MICHAEL NARRATOR

With the increase of partying, came an increase in sexually transmitted diseases, not only in the Gay Community but also in the Straight Community. In those days, people went to the bar not only to have a drink and visit but also to find a "one night stand," sometimes each night of the week, with whom to go home. Let's take a visit to the Howard Brown Clinic, created by the Gay Community to help serve the needs of the community which the straight community was not yet so eagerly ready to do. Gregory comes down with what ends up being an infection, not sexually transmitted, but all five of the six "partners" involved in this non-magnanimous relationship go to the clinic to get checked out. Gregory's other love lives in Boston so he does not need an exam.

SETTING

The scene opens in a clinic with a few rows of chairs and a reception desk. Furnished in a somewhat makeshift manner and in the style of the day. There is a door leading off to the doctor's offices. Gregory and Michael along with Barbara, Robert, Greg B., are seated waiting for their appointment. The dialogue is meant to show the beginnings of sexual freedom, many one night stands, and the increasing risk of STD's.

MUSIC

Everyone arrives at the clinic including a few others already in the waiting room. Music comes up and backs an energetic TAP DANCE number showing off all the usual route steps and athleticism. The scene ends with everyone flopping back into their seats as the receptionist announces:

RECEPTIONIST

The doctor is ready to see the Horvich/Maire group now.

ACT TWO SCENE THREE
HIV/AIDS
(1980's)

SETTING

The group slowly reassembles in the waiting room and authentic, live TV coverage comes up on a large screen TV talking about the new "Gay Disease," the new "Gay Cancer." Then shifts to some interviews with people affected by HIV/AIDS showing just how severe the disease can be. The presentation continues on to a point where

many people are being diagnosed, many are dying, there still is no
cure, it is now realized that the epidemic is not only affecting Gays.

MUSIC

Pensive, foreboding, sad.

ACT TWO SCENE FOUR
I Love You – II

(1990's)

OLD MAN NARRATOR

Let's skip ahead to the 90's. Gregory and Michael have been living
with each other in a committed relationship for close to fifteen years
and have created a beautiful, welcoming, comfortable home for
themselves.

SETTING

Their discussion in the living room shows them as a loving, settled
couple. Gregory is working as a counselor for people with
developmental difficulties and living in a group residence and
Michael is teaching fourth grade in a Chicago suburb school system.

GREGORY AND MICHAEL DIALOGUE: (TBD)

They sing a song about their love, their life, and spending time together. Ballad?

ACT TWO SCENE FIVE
Second Gay March on Washington D.C.
(1993)

SETTING

(In front of curtain, lights come up on a video or slide show of the march including newspaper headlines touting statistics of attendance etc.)

OLD MICHAEL NARRATOR DIALOGUE: (TBD)

During the slide show, gives some background on the march like purpose and number of people attending.

ACT TWO SCENE SIX
Walk Across: Gay Pride Parade
(2000's)

SETTING

Continues in front of curtain. Similar to previous walk around but this time it is apparent that the parade of the 90' has progressed since the first one in the 70'.s It is a lot bigger, more energetic, more celebratory, friendlier supportive crowds watching, less of a police presence, many famous "brand "products with floats . Marchers enter stage right, cross, exit stage left, drop prop or costume, cross behind curtain, pick up new prop or costume, enter again. Slow black out.)

MUSIC

Peppy, march, parade type music.

ACT TWO SCENE SEVEN
Vermont Civil Union
(2000)

SETTING

New England Cottage by a stream. A rainbow is in the sky. The multi-generation, Vermontian, older woman Justice of the Peace, Elizabeth performs the marriage ceremony in her living room which is dark, over upholstered, warm, inviting, fire in fireplace. Michael and Gregory have brought a bottle of wine, Elizabeth has baked cookies.

MUSIC

The ceremony could be sung by Elizabeth. Perhaps operatic reflecting the solemnity of the occasion and the age of the woman.

GREGORY/MICHAEL/ELIZABETH DIALOGUE (TBD)

Before, during, and after the ceremony?

INTERMISSION

ALZHEIMER'S

A MUSICAL
LOVE STORY

Love, Life, & Liberation

By Michael A. Horvich & Gregory L. Maire

WORKING TITLES

GREGORY:

An Alzheimer's
LOVE STORY

Love, Life, & Liberation

By Michael A. Horvich & Gregory L. Maire

ACT III

ALZHEIMER'S

A MUSICAL LOVE STORY

Love, Life, & Liberation

By Michael A. Horvich & Gregory L. Maire

WORKING TITLES

GREGORY:

An Alzheimer's LOVE STORY

Love, Life, & Liberation

By Michael A. Horvich & Gregory L. Maire

ACT THREE SCENE ONE
The Diagnosis
(2003)

Sound in the dark of a noise cancelling machine.(Sound of noise cancelling machine fades. Brief silence then

NURSE *(in darkness)*

Mr. Maire, Mr. Horvich … the doctor will see you now. This way please …

SETTING

When lights come up Instant all-on stage lights. White. So white that it almost hurts to look at it. Everything on stage is in white: small center cubical, walls, picture in frame on wall, desk, doctor's chair, two client chairs, flowers on desk, telephone, doctor's patient file, pens and pencils in holder, pen in doctor's hand. Doctor in white lab coat and pants is seated behind the desk slightly downstage left. Gregory (55 years old) and Michael (58 years old) in white jeans and shirts are seated across from the doctor slightly upstage right. ALL STARK WHITE.

DOCTOR

(While well-meaning and kind, you can tell he is uncomfortable giving his findings and seems to be meandering and circling around whatever comes to his mind that he thinks he probably should be saying ... or maybe not! Addressing Michael. Ignores Gregory through entire scene. Hesitates as though gathering his thoughts. Not meant to portray the doctor as a buffoon but rather uncomfortable and inept in "bedside manner.")

As you know the diagnosis of Dementia, most likely Alzheimer's, will help us understand what has been going on with you ... and what we can expect as the disease progresses ... *(somewhat pensive and to himself)* ... progresses ... funny use of the term.

There are at least ten diseases related to and/or with symptoms we could call ... Dementia. *(Rattles them off rapidly)* These include Alzheimer's, Vascular, Lewy Bodies, Parkinson's, Frontotemporal, Creutzfeldt-Jakob, Huntington's, Wernicke-Korsakoff, and of course Dementia due to just good old (hesitates) ... old age.

They are all incurable, *(Almost to himself)* I guess that's the BAD news.

The GOOD news is that this is not a death sentence. A person can live a long, productive life with the disease. *(Addressing Michael)* With the support of family, friends, his medical team and a willingness and ability to change as the disease progresses ... *(almost to himself)* there is that word again ... progress ... *(Back to addressing Michael.)*

Of course, we cannot tell for sure that he has Alzheimer's and won't be able to until we do an autopsy *(makes a face in a "should I have said that way) if you want one after death … (almost to himself) …* should we be talking about this?

And by calling it Alzheimer's *(even if it isn't)* it will simplify explaining the situation to the people in your life and to insurance companies as well.

We have ruled out what is NOT causing what is going on here … which <u>could be</u> curable: *(rattles them off rapidly)* no vitamin B deficiency, no strokes or TAI's, no Delirium, no Normal Pressure Hydrocephalus, no problems with vision or hearing, no disorders of the heart or lungs, no liver or kidney disease, no hormone disruption, no infections, and no cancer. Isn't the body an amazing thing?

So that is the GOOD NEWS … but it points to the BAD NEWS that your diagnosis is Dementia, most likely Alzheimer's Disease, which is progressive and incurable *(shoulder shrug, head tip.)*

(The doctor stands up to signal that the visit is over.)

Let's follow up in six months, if you need anything be sure to call my office. Thank you, Mr. Horvich, … *(then as an afterthought)* Mr. Maire.

As Gregory and Michael stand to leave

the lights fade out and to black. They are picked up in warmer spots

on a dark stage.

MICHAEL

Wow! At least we now understand what's been happening to us. Together we WILL get through this! And you know what? … I … LOVE … YOU … MORE … THAN … EVER!

They hug and melt into each other's arms.

ACT THREE SCENE TWO
MORE THAN EVER
(2005)

SETTING

Doctor's office disappears leaving Gregory and Michael stage center in a romantic spotlight.

MUSIC

A love song in which Gregory and Michael continue to fall in love despite the diagnosis of Dementia most likely Alzheimer's. A love song in which they reaffirm their love for each other in the face of this insidious, devastating disease.

Could have some information about Dementia as the symptoms and Alzheimer's as the disease. Could include learning to live day by day, not letting the diagnosis be a death sentence, closing the business and traveling the country and the world. Could be a slide show or WALK ACROSS.

ACT THREE SCENE THREE
LIVING WITH ALZHEIMER'S
(2007)

SETTING

Gregory at his desk. His behaviors show how he is losing skills. Possibly forgets how to use a newspaper, colors with wrong side of crayon, doesn't know how to drink from his mug, crumbles cookie by accident in too strong of a hand hold, spills his water glass. Calls "MICHAEL, I you're your help! MICHAEL, MICHAEL? "

MUSIC

Lyrics from Person With Dementia (PWD,) discusses some of the losses and compensations, skills come and go and return only to eventually disappear, frustration, fears.

Lyrics from Person Loving PWD, discusses losses, fears, frustrations, trying to deal with respect, etc Solos and Duet about issues of change for the couple.

ACT THREE SCENE FOUR
LIVING WITH MORE ALZHEIMER'S
(2011)

SETTING

A series of vignettes, serious and funny scenes the result of the disease. ***(TBD)***

MUSIC

Circus Music? Overture music reprise?

ACT THREE SCENE FIVE
WALK ACROSS—GREGORY'S DECLINE (2013)

SETTING

Michael and Gregory cross stage several times demonstrating Gregory's decline. Set Michael and Gregory arriving in the garden behind a fence at Lieberman. A sign informs that it is a Memory Care Facility.

1. *Arriving in garden together normally. Gregory is engaged.*
2. *Arriving slowly with Michael holding Gregory's hand guiding him. Gregory still engaged.*

3. *Walking Michael ahead of Gregory, Michael turns back to grab Gregory to guide him. Gregory looks less engaged and a little unsure of his walking.*

4. *Walking Michael with no Gregory, turns, goes back to get Gregory, now minimally engaged and very slow.*

5. *Michael pushing Gregory in a wheel chair, Gregory fairly unengaged.*

MUSIC

To music mostly "heavy" and sad with feeling of progression of disease and foreboding future

ACT THREE SCENE SIX
HOW CAN I GO ON?
(2014)

SETTING

Michael walks back into garden alone, having dropped Gregory off, and sings.

MUSIC

Retrospective, sad ballad.

ACT IV

ALZHEIMER'S
A MUSICAL LOVE STORY
Love, Life, & Liberation
By Michael A. Horvich & Gregory L. Maire

WORKING TITLES

GREGORY:
An Alzheimer's LOVE STORY
Love, Life, & Liberation
By Michael A. Horvich & Gregory L. Maire

ACT FOUR SCENE ONE
Song Without Words
(2014)

Michael pushing Gregory in a wheel chair across the stage as the "Lieberman Garden" moves in a diorama past them. Gregory is enjoying the fresh air and both Michael and Gregory are very much in the "Here and Now."

Michael pauses half way across stage and Gregory mumbles he wants Michael's attention. Gregory reaches for Michael's hand and holds it tight. Gregory is at the same time happy and sad and full of love for Michael.

Gregory proceeds to sing a beautiful love song to Michael, none of which is understandable, none of which has any content, only connectors and hesitations and sighs and looking for words but none arrive or mixed, unrelated words. Gregory slowly gets frustrated but Michael leans in, kisses Gregory on the forehead and says, "I know, I know." This cheers Gregory up as he finishes his love song.

MUSIC
Love song but words make no sense.

✳✳✳

ACT FOUR SCENE TWO
Same Sex Marriage in Illinois and the U.S.
(2014/15)

SETTING

On back wall, a newspaper announcing "Same Sex Marriage Passes Court." Black stage with couples bathed in spotlights. A ballet of man/woman, man/man, woman/woman couples. Two pairs of each of above representing gay men, lesbians, and transsexuals. Sexes of participants very obvious as in beards for men and long hair/breasts for women.

MUSIC

Formal ballet

COSTUMES

Man/man—Tuxedos

Man/man—Tuxedo & wedding dress

Woman/woman—Wedding dresses

Woman/woman—Tuxedo & wedding dress

Man/woman—Tuxedo and wedding dress

Man/woman-Wedding dress and tuxedo

DIALOGUE TBD: OLD MICHAEL NARRATOR

Relates that while Gregory and Michael have a civil union in Vermont (which amounts to no protections outside of Vermont, just a reaffirmation of their love for each other.) Recaps governmental acclaims about Gay Marriage, but this exciting news comes a little late for them.

Ballet shows all variation of people in love, interacting, happy. Ballet ends with Gregory and Micha sitting together at the Lieberman Memory Care facility with Gregory in state of Dementita "unavailability."

ACT FOUR SCENE THREE
Sharing Love
(2014)

SETTING

Scene opens at Lieberman Memory Care Facility. Gregory's empty bedroom.

A CNA wheels Gregory into the room in a downstage center spot (gently soft quality of light) on an otherwise black stage. Another CNA moves a bedside table and leaves it just behind and to stage left of Gregory.

Gregory is unavailable and looks like he is sleeping. Covered with a blanket and a pillow tucked under his head which tilts gently to stage left. He is holding Peaceful the Bear.

Michael enters upstage right, crosses left and down, and stops short of approaching Gregory who is sleeping.

MUSIC

Michael sings a song of joy with sorrow, hope with despair, laughter with tears, love with pain, fears with confidence. They have been dealing with Dementia for close to twelve years. Michael sings of what he misses as Gregory slowly loses his abilities.

The music continues as a full, powerful instrumental. Quietly in the beginning and growing and growing as Michael moves a chair next to Gregory, stage, gently touching Gregory's face with his right hand. Music stops as Gregory wakes up, Michael says "hello" with his facial and shoulder gesture. Gregory recognizes (in a removed way) that Michael is there to visit.

Michael removes and folds the blanket hanging it over the back of the chair. He next picks up Peaceful from Gregory's arms and puts him on Gregory's wheelchair footrest.

Reprise of music picks up again as Michael proceeds to do things that demonstrate his love for Gregory and Gregory in his "unavailable way" accepts and acknowledges the gestures of gentle love, visible to the audience

Michael rubs Gregory's shoulders from Gregory's stage left. Gregory shows contentment at the rub. Michael kisses Gregory on the mouth and Gregory receives the kiss but not with much energy. Next Michael brushes Gregory's hair. Michael picks up a glass of water and helps Gregory drink. Michael dries Gregory's mouth with a napkin. Then Michael leans over and hugs Gregory. Perhaps you can see Michael's shoulders heave with a sad sigh. Michael sits down and takes Gregory's hand and rubs his own (Michael's) head lovingly.

Gregory indicates in a removed way, by sitting a little forward, looking at Michael to stage left and inclining his head towards Michael, that Gregory wants another kiss. Michael stands and leans in and gives him one. Then breaks kiss just a little to stare into Gregory's eyes and then leans in to continue the kiss. Michael again hugs Gregory and the two gently rocking until the end of the music. Slowly the lights fade to black.

ACT FOUR SCENE FOUR
RIP Gregory Maire

(October 4, 2015)

Up with intense white, almost blinding in Gregory's stark room at Lieberman Memory Care facility, for death scene. Gregory is in bed with covers up to his neck, his arms are outside the covers and he is holding Peaceful. Michael sits on a chair next to the bed close to Gregory saying his final goodbyes.

MUSIC

Michael begins the "Good Bye" song, expressing thoughts and feelings for himself as well as for Gregory since Gregory no longer has language. (Could be a duet with Gregory "regaining" language with "magical realism." Slowly during the song, Gregory gets weaker and weaker, the spot light on Gregory gets brighter and brighter. The spot light on Michael gets dimmer and dimmer. Eventually by the end of the song, Gregory is bathed on intense white, Michael is not visible, and then BLACK OUT.

ACT FOUR SCENE FIVE
Possibility A

A Monologue: The Heart Sutra

(2015)

SETTING

Michael sitting on a bench. The backdrop is of a beautiful fall forest at sunset with the light's yellow, orange, and red playing of the trees and leaves. Michael is staring at a piece of paper which he is holding in his hand. He addresses the audience. (Must be done in a way that helps the audience to clearly understand this complicated notion of the Buddhist Heart Sutra.)

MICHAEL

Several times towards the end I encouraged Gregory to "leave us" when he was ready. I did not want him to linger thinking I needed him to stay so I told him, "I will miss you and be ever so sad, but I will be OK and you will be OK too!

(Michael begins to get choked up. He pats the place on the bench next to him, gains his composure, and continues.)

The HEART SUTRA is a BUDDHIST scripture. I love the Buddhist Monk, Thich Nhat Hanh's translation and explanation.

This empty piece of paper sums it up and it has helped me get past the overwhelming grief that I feel with Gregory's death.

No one thing can exist without the things that make it up. So, this piece of paper is made up of the wood of the tree from which it was made, but also the sunshine it took to grow the tree, the rain that watered the tree, the logger who logged the tree, the parents that gave birth to the logger, the wheat that fed the logger, the manufacturer who processed the paper, the stationary store that sold the paper, and finally me, who purchased the paper.

I could go on, but you get the point, this piece of paper does not have its own identity, it is made up of everything that surrounded its growth, manufacture, and eventually the sale and the purchasing of it.

With Thich Nhat Hanh's explanation I now understand that **no single item has its own unique, identity.** Everything exists because of everything else which brought it into being.

I am part of this piece of paper also because I have written on it … and so does Gregory since he was part of my life and part of my writing and my poetry.

Without Gregory, and all experiences and people who have walked across my path since the day I was born, I would not be the Michael I am!

One way to be in touch with the Heart Sutra is the chant: Gate, Gate, Paragate, Parasamgate. Bodhi. Svatwa.

Translated: Gone. Gone. We are all gone. To the other side, where we can seek enlightenment. So be it!

As long as I continue to exist, Gregory exists. As long as his name is spoken, and he is remembered, and loved … he exists.

As long as I breathe the air, I am breathing the same air Gregory used to breathe. I am still hugged by Gregory, my lips are still kissed by his lips, I drift off to sleep at night as we still embrace each other with admiration, fondness, love, and respect!

There is no life and there is no death. There just is!

My poet friend Kate Swaffer, who I met on Facebook and who lives well with Dementia/ Alzheimer's in Australia, wrote this poem:

> Remember when the time comes
> Breathe in very deep
> Take my very last breath
> And make it your own.

When Gregory died, I did just that. I kissed him, sat next to him, and breathed in deeply. So now I am not only me, but I am also a bit more of Gregory … and who knows … where ever Gregory is … perhaps he is also a bit more of me?

(Gregory slowly "materializes" on the bench next to me.)

When I left Gregory for the final time, I stopped briefly before getting into my car. What was I feeling? *(pause)*

First, I felt immense sorrow but right next to that I felt freedom. I felt that the hole which had been ripped in my heart and chest over the last twelve years, could now begin to heal.

I felt happiness for Gregory. In one moment, the moment he died, the Alzheimer's disappeared, puff, like smoke in the air.

Gregory was free from the debilitating disease and so was I.

Gregory was full again, no longer weighed down by the loss of words, the loss of abilities, the loss of quality of life. He could move on now, happiness in his heart.

I was full again, no longer weighed down by watching my lover, my best friend, my soul mate, my husband slowly disappears. I could move on now, happiness in my heart.

The scene dissolves into the next one.

]
ACT FOUR SCENE FIVE
Possibility B

A Lament of Joy
(2015)

SETTING

A slide montage of real life Gregory and Michael, arm and arm, from when they first met through the Dementia/Alzheimer's years and up to Gregory's death.

MUSIC

"Happiness is Here and Now:" from Plum Village by Vietnamese Monk Thich Nhat Hanh.
Possibly projected on rear wall?

GREGORY
Happiness is here and now.
I have dropped my worries.
Nothing to do. Nowhere to go.
There's no need for hurry.

MICHAEL
Happiness is here and now.
I have dropped my worries.
Something to do. **Somewhere** to go.
But, there's **no need for hurry.**

GREGORY & MICHAEL
Happiness is here and now.
Happiness is here and now.
I have dropped my worries.
I have dropped my worries.
Nothing to do. Nowhere to go
Something to do. Somewhere to go.
There's no need for hurry.
There's no need for hurry.

The Greek Chorus slowly joins in singing with love as Gregory and Michael pause. Music gets louder and more dynamic and louder and louder.

Happiness is here and now.
We have dropped our worries.

Nothing to do. Nowhere to go.
There's no need for hurry.

Happiness is here and now.
We have dropped our worries.
Something to do. Somewhere to go.
But, there's no need for hurry.

ACT FOUR SCENE SIX
Possibility A
A Lament of Joy

(2015)

MUSIC

Something like <u>Priscilla Queen of Desert</u> 's "True Color" or an original piece that is upbeat and hopeful and loving. Ability to bring audience to a comfortable place after a "roller coaster ride" with Dementia/Alzheimer's experience.

SETTING

During entire show, scenes have changed with large placards moving slowly across stage showing calendar/year, title of scene, photo, and/or newspaper headlines. As placard moved across stage, new scene was being set in dark behind, then lights up on scene.

For the finale, all scene change placards are lowered or move onto stage, and go through a dynamic, intense, colorful light show which ends in a cross-stage rainbow.

ACT FOUR SCENE SIX
Possibility B

If I Knew Then

(2015)

MUSIC

Deals with looking back and looking forward. In the style of an opera quartet and then joined by the chorus.

From his point of view, older Michael sings, "If I knew then what I know now." Younger Michael joins stage and from his point of view sings, "If I could know now what I will know then." They sing a duet.

From his point of view, older Gregory sings, "If I could know then what I know now." Younger Gregory joins stage and from his point of view sings, "If I could know now what I will know then."

They sing a duet.

Song ends with a quartet, everyone singing at same time but with various important points of view from the four people coming into focus through the piece.

Chorus joins stage for a rousing end.

CURTAIN & BOWS

APPENDICES

ALZHEIMER'S
A MUSICAL LOVE STORY
Love, Life, & Liberation
By Michael A. Horvich & Gregory L. Maire

WORKING TITLES

GREGORY:
An Alzheimer's LOVE STORY
Love, Life, & Liberation
By Michael A. Horvich & Gregory L. Maire

APPENDICES:

APPENDIX:
MEET MICHAEL

Younger Michael
Age 5

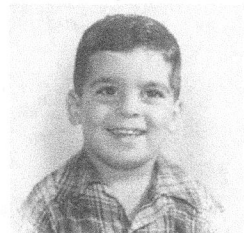

Older Michael
Age 75

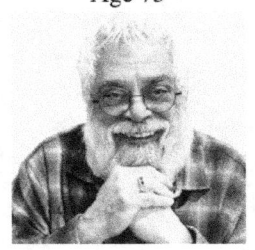

Michael's Family
Adeline RIP 2010, Michael BORN 1945
Libbe RIP 2020, Louis RIP 2005

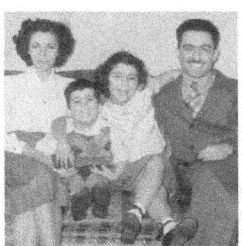

Michael's Gregory
RIP 10/04/2015

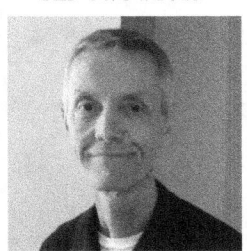

Michael's Pets
Emma & Gigi

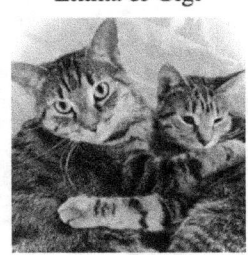

APPENDIX:
ABOUT MICHAEL short version

Michael A. Horvich
Michael has been called a "Renaissance Man."

Michael is an educator, motivational speaker, story-teller, writer, poet, photographer, blogger, artist, jeweler, book binder, lecturer, actor, supernumerary, collector, museum curator, flea circus ring master, and was a Dementia/Alzheimer's caregiver partner for his partner Gregory Maire (RIP 2015.)

He won two Fellowships in Gifted Education from the State of Illinois, a Performing Arts Grant from the City of Chicago for "Maybe the Clown and His Back Pocket Review, and a two-week Competitive Application Residency in creative non-fiction writing at The Ragdale Foundation in Lake Forest, Illinois.

Michael's Museum: A Curious Collection of Tiny Treasures, a folk-art collection of over 105 collections was installed as a permanent exhibit at The Chicago Children's Museum on Navy Pier in May, 2011.

He has been a Supernumerary, an acting extra, at Lyric Opera of Chicago in 20 operas over a period of 13 years.

He and his life partner Gregory Maire (RIP,) are the subject of "ALZHEIMER'S: A Love Story," which has been accepted nationally and internationally by 90+ film festivals and has won 35+ awards. The documentary can be seen on with the link on Michael's website.

He has self-published 13 books of poetry, memoirs, philosophy, fiction; and on Michael's Museum, Alzheimer's support, LGBTQ Issues, and grief support.

APPENDIX:
ABOUT MICHAEL long version

Michael A. Horvich

One rare piece that was inherited and has provenance is a treasure.
One rare piece that you bought and has provenance is a treasure.
Collections that consist of rare pieces and have provenance will be
welcome at auctions and by dealers. Provenance is a written history
or pedigree of a piece

The Collector's Dilemma. Jeanne Siegel. 2006.

• • •

This is a written history of Michael A. Horvich, Evanston, Illinois,
Born March 27, 1945.

Michael received his BA in Liberal Arts and Sciences from the
University of Illinois at Urbana/Champaign in conjunction with
studies done at Hunter College in New York City. He received his
MA as an Educational Generalist in the area of Gifted Education from
the National Lewis University in Evanston. He did his Advanced
Certificate work and ABD (all but doctoral dissertation) in the area of
Educational Supervision and Administration at the University of
Illinois.

He worked in a residential treatment research center with children in
trouble with the law, helped found a school for children diagnosed
with Autism, directed a day camp, and taught pre-school children and
teenagers with developmental disabilities.

In the public school setting he taught fourth and fifth grades, junior
high Spanish, and created as well as served as administrator for the

district wide program for Gifted Education students in Glenview Schools #34. Michael has published about Talented and Gifted Education in several educational journals.

He was an adjunct faculty member of National Lewis University, presented workshops and taught courses in Gifted Education for the State of Illinois Department of Education, had several articles published in educational journals, and twice was awarded a State of Illinois Fellowship in Gifted Education.

He received a grant from the Chicago Council on Fine Arts for his "Maybe-the-Clown and His Back Pocket Review," which was performed all around Chicago including public schools, on the Michigan Avenue Bridge, on the steps of the Art Institute, at Lincoln Park Zoo, and elsewhere.

His Book Arts abilities were presented in a show at the Jane Adams Hull House in Chicago and his photographs and jewelry have been part of silent auctions at several charitable foundations.

As a Supernumerary with The Lyric Opera of Chicago, he was an acting-extra for fifteen years and appeared in over twenty operas.

In 1999, after thirty years as an educator, Michael retired to pursue other avenues of creativity. Since then, he has been more than active as a speaker, story teller, writer, poet, photographer, blogger, artist, jeweler, lecturer, actor, supernumerary, museum curator, flea circus ring master, philanthropist, and Dementia/Alzheimer's caregiver partner for his life partner Gregory Maire (RIP 2015)

Michael is a collector of collections. His miniature book collection has been on display at the Glenview and Evanston Public Libraries. His collection of North American Indian Arts and Crafts miniatures has been on display at both libraries as well as at the Mitchell Indian Museum in Evanston.

His life partner Gregory, was diagnosed in 2003 with Dementia, most likely Alzheimer's Disease. Gregory lived with the disease for twelve years, was able to be at home for most of that time, and died in 2015.

In 2010 Michael won, by competitive competition, a residency in Creative Non-Fiction at The Ragdale Foundation in Lake Forest, IL.

He created and was curator of Michael's Museum, a private collection located in his home, of hundreds of thousands of pieces grouped into over 105 collections of small things: miniatures, curiosities, discoverings, trinkets, oddities, artifacts, antiquities, and collectibles.

Michael's Museum was given to, and has been a permanent exhibit at the Chicago Children's Museum on Navy Pier since May of 2011. Michael is now Curator Emiratis of this very popular exhibit which is visited by more than half a million people a year.

Michael maintained a writer's BLOG. One dealing with Alzheimer's Disease is no longer active but contains many interesting and useful pieces in archive. The other is his writer's BLOG. While both BLOGS are inactive, they have archived a lot of useful material.

Shortly before Gregory's death in 2015, a 15-minute documentary, "ALZHEIMER'S: A Love Story," was made. It follows Gregory and Michael for a week, with Gregory having lived at the Lieberman Mental Health Facility for approximately one year.

The documentary has been accepted by more than 90 film festivals in the U.S. and around the world and has won over 30 awards including two at the American Pavilion at the Cannes Film Festival.

As the documentary is watched, the fact that it deals with a same-sex couple and Alzheimer's Disease begins to disappear. What emerges is a love story about any two people who love each other and what they face during a catastrophic, long-term illness. The story he tells provides hope in what could be a hopeless situation!

Following that, Michael began professionally speaking about such issues as Alzheimer's Disease, Healthy Grieving, and LGBTQ Issues to a wide variety of groups including: Northshore University Health Care System Division of Palliative Care and Hospice, United Methodist Church of LaGrange Illinois, University of Chicago Middle School Students, Lieberman Center for Health and Rehabilitation, Sherman Plaza Book and Social Club, Dementia Alliance International of Australia, and Pritzker School of Medicine.

He has also made presentations for Northwestern University Kellogg Graduate School of Business, Great Lakes Alzheimer's Association, Battle Creek Congregational Church, 33rd Annual Alzheimer's

Disease International Convention, Proud Seniors of Athens Greece, the Chicago LGBTQ Center on Halsted, DePaul University, Northwestern University Medical Center, Evanston Art Center, and the Prime Timers Men's Group of Chicago.

During 2019, Michael made the opening key-note for 1,500 attendees and facilitated a break-out group for over 100 people in "The Dimensions of Love and Grief" at the Mayo Clinic and Minnesota-North Dakota Alzheimer's Association Conference which took place in St. Paul. While there, he was part of a program on NPR dealing with Alzheimer's Disease.

Michael and Gregory are co-founders of La Casa Norte's More Than Ever Education Fund, in memory of Gregory, which since 2015 has raised over $250,000 to support youth confronting homelessness pursue their educational degrees.

He lives in Evanston with his cats Emma and Gigi

So far, Michael has self-published thirteen books:
- POETRY: Sit with Me A While, Sit with Me A While Longer, and Sit with Me Another While Longer
- FICTION: Counting Down the Yardstick
- PHILOSOPHY: A Pondering: Thoughts on Thinking
- ALZHEIMER'S: Gyroscope: An Alzheimer's Love Story
- COLLECTIONS: Michael's Museum: A Curious Collection of Tiny Treasures: Volume 1—The Story, Volume II—The Photographs
- MEMOIRS: The Museum of Michael's Mind Volume One and Two
- LGBTQ STORIES: Written for Prism & Pen—Volume One and Two
- GRIEVING: Good Grief: Grieve Correctly—Do It your Own Way!
- AN ALZHEIMER'S LOVE STORY: A Preparation and Proposal

APPENDIX:
FOLLOW MICHAEL

www.horvich.com

*He shares many of his interests
with links on his website.*

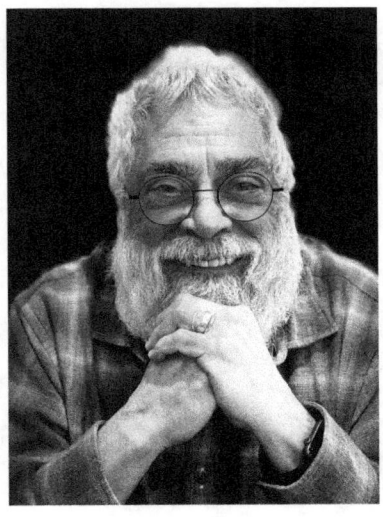

✳✳✳

APPENDIX:
BOOKS BY MICHAEL

Some of Michael's books are available at:
www.amazon.com
www.barnesandnoble.com

All of Michael's books are available at:
www.lulu.com

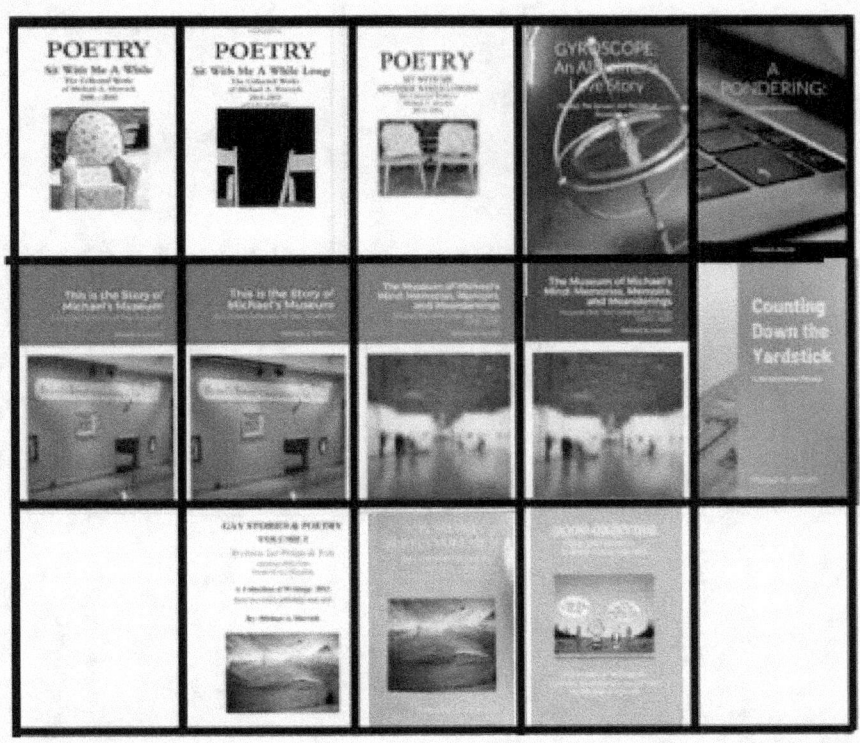

This is the Story of Michael's Museum

A Curious Collection of Tiny Treasures

Michael A. Horvich

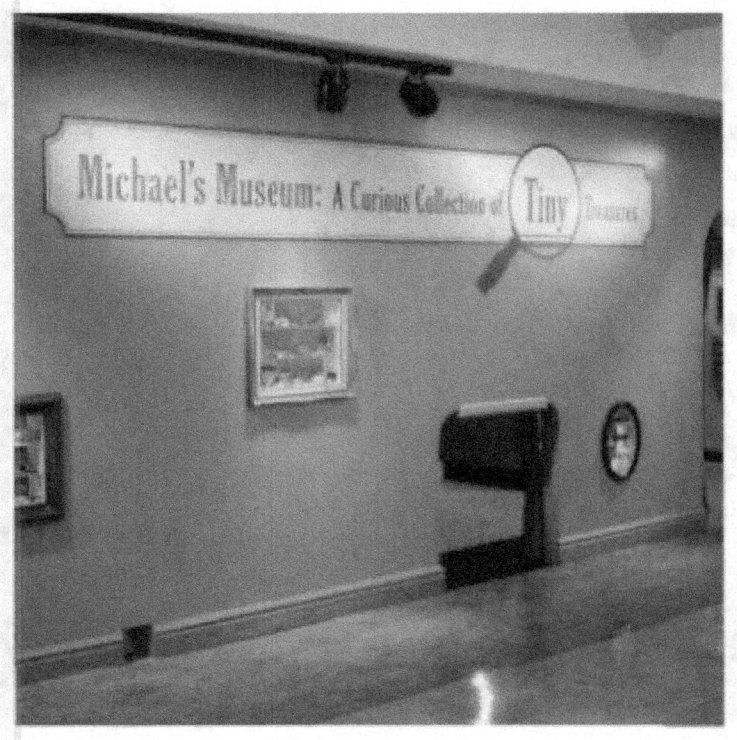

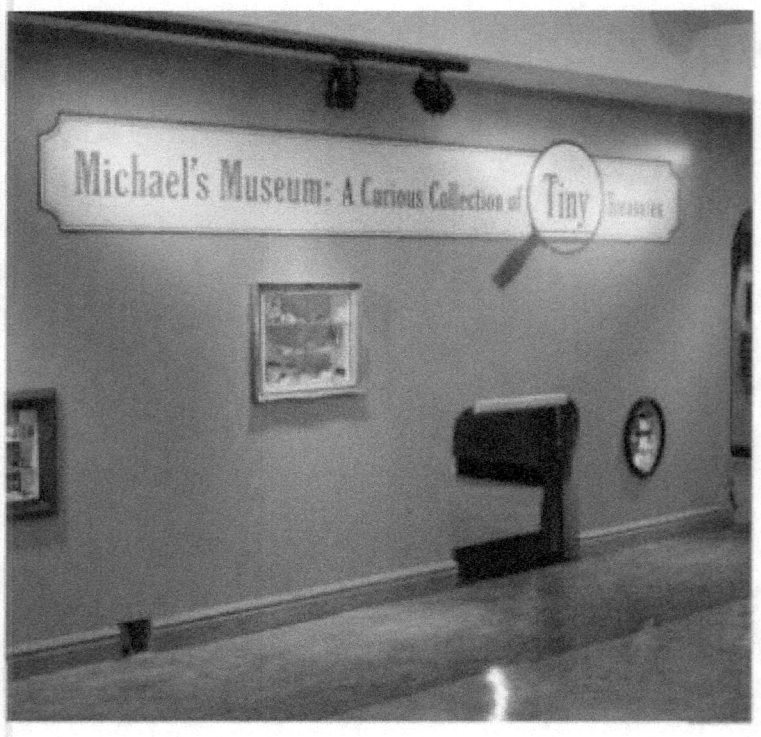

Counting Down the Yardstick

A Reincarnation Memoir

Michael A. Horvich

POETRY

Sit With Me A While

The Collected Works
of Michael A. Horvich
2000 - 2010

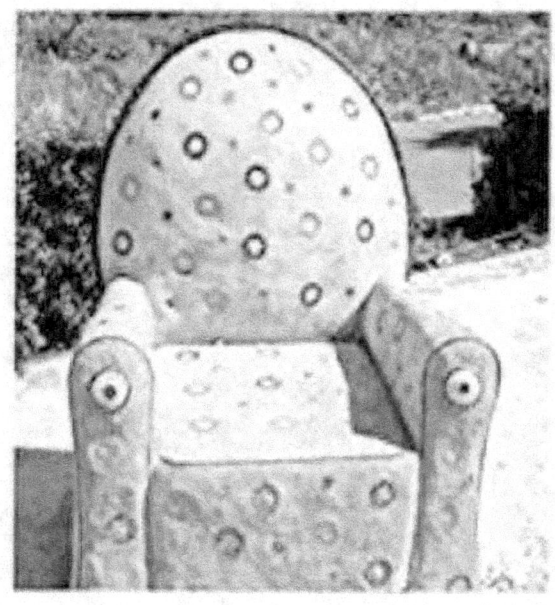

POETRY

Sit With Me A While Longer

The Collected Works
of Michael A. Horvich
2011-2013

and a few earlier ones

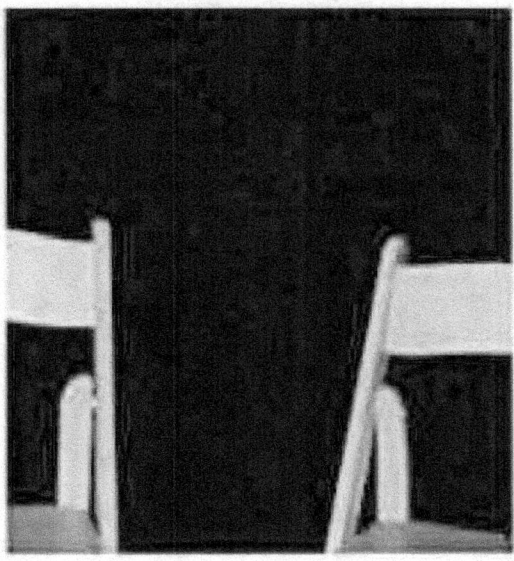

POETRY

SIT WITH ME
ANOTHER WHILE LONGER

The Collected Works of
Michael A. Horvich
2013-2021

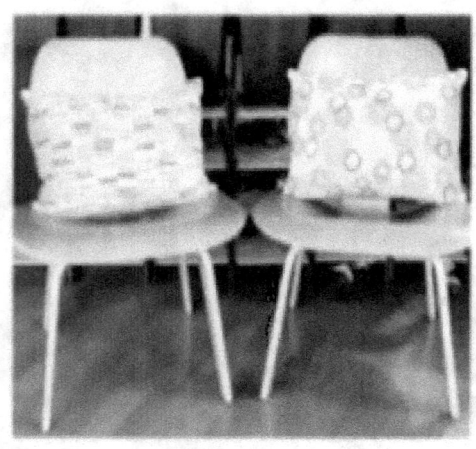

The Museum of Michael's Mind: Memories, Memoirs, and Meanderings
Volume One: The Collected Writings 2005–2015

Michael A. Horvich

The Museum of Michael's Mind: Memories, Memoirs, and Meandersings

Volume Two: The Collected Writings
2016–2020

Michael A. Horvich

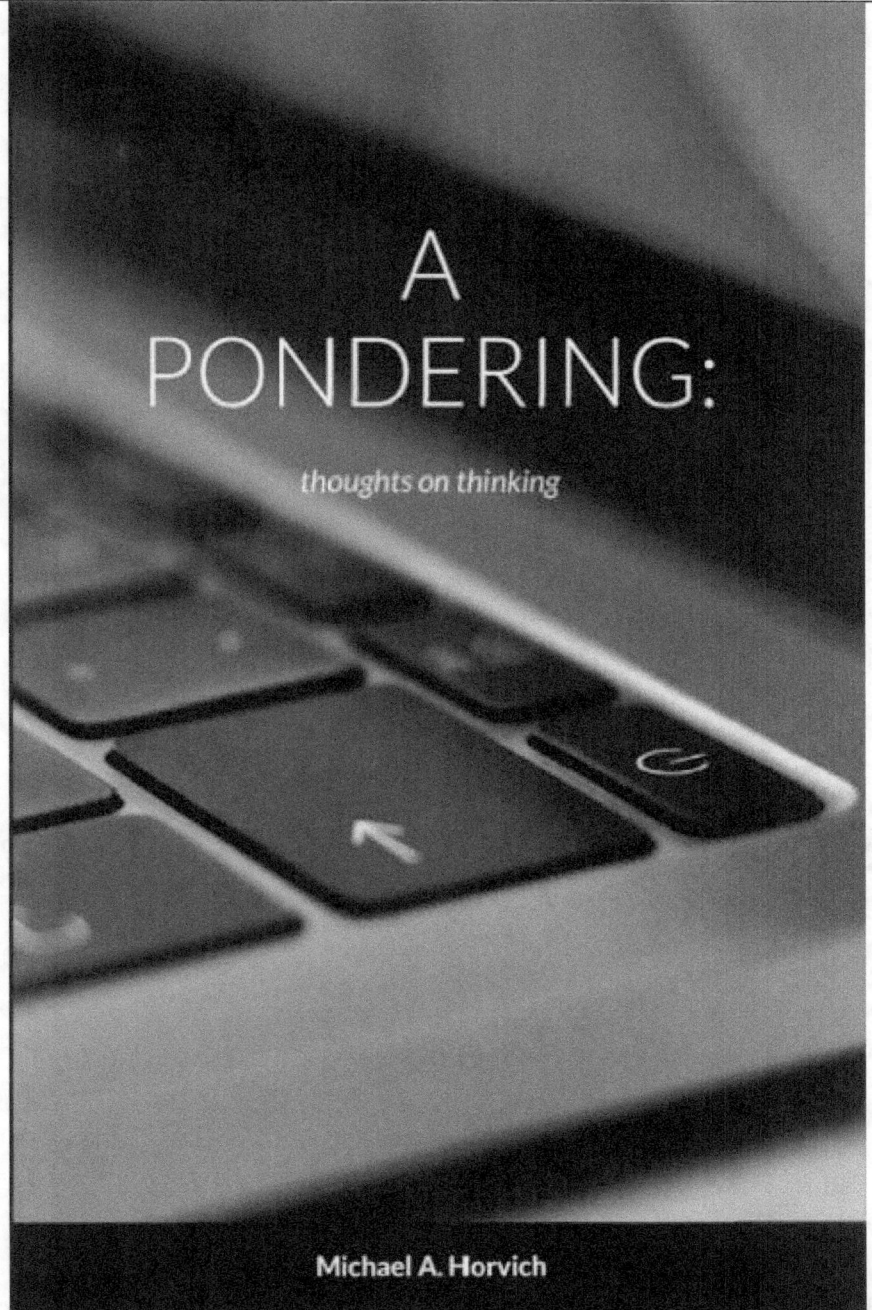

A PONDERING:

thoughts on thinking

Michael A. Horvich

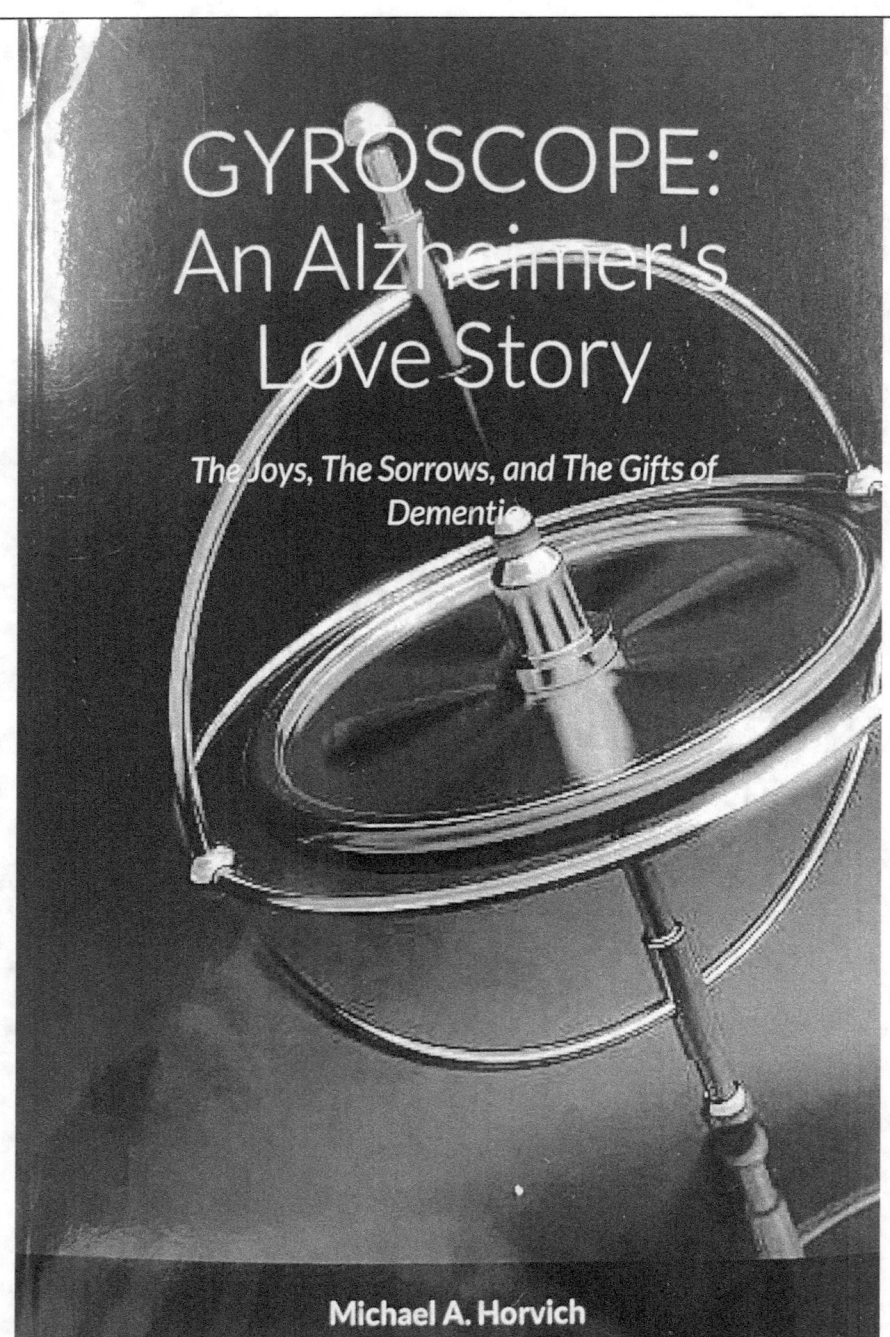

GYROSCOPE:
An Alzheimer's
Love Story

*The Joys, The Sorrows, and The Gifts of
Dementia*

Michael A. Horvich

GAY STORIES & POETRY VOLUME I

Written for Prism & Pen

Amplifying LGBTQ Voices

Through The Art of Storytelling

A Collection of Writings: 2022

Some previously published some new

By: Michael A. Horvich

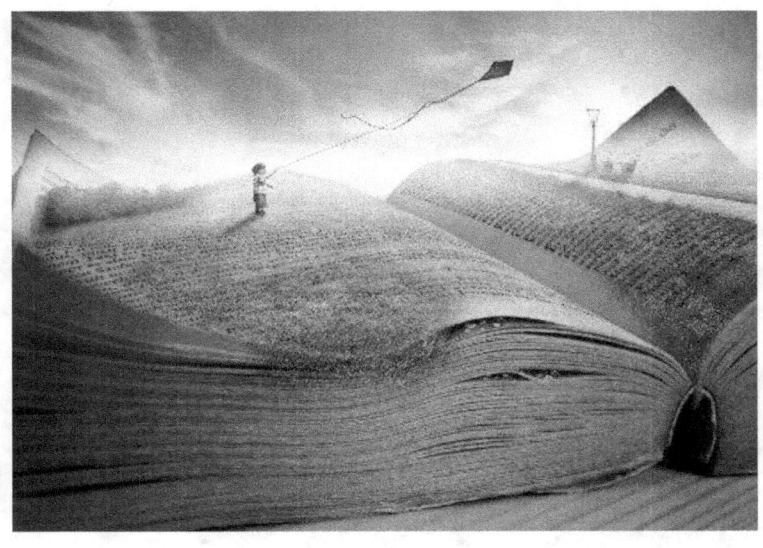

GAY STORIES & POETRY
VOLUME II

Written for Prism & Pen

Amplifying LGBTQ Voices

Through The Art of Storytelling

A Collection of Writings: 2023

Some previously published some new

By: Michael A. Horvich

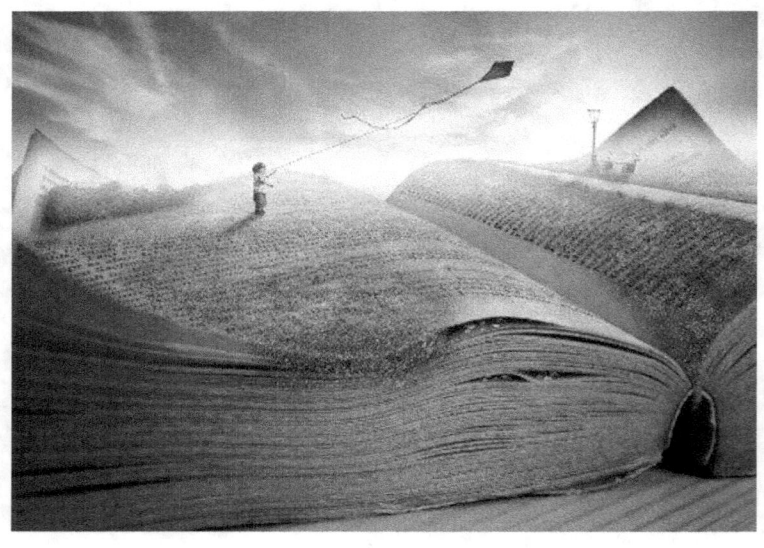

GOOD GRIEVING

Doing grief correctly…by doing it your own way!

A Collection of Writings on Grieving the Death of a Loved One

By: Michael A. Horvich

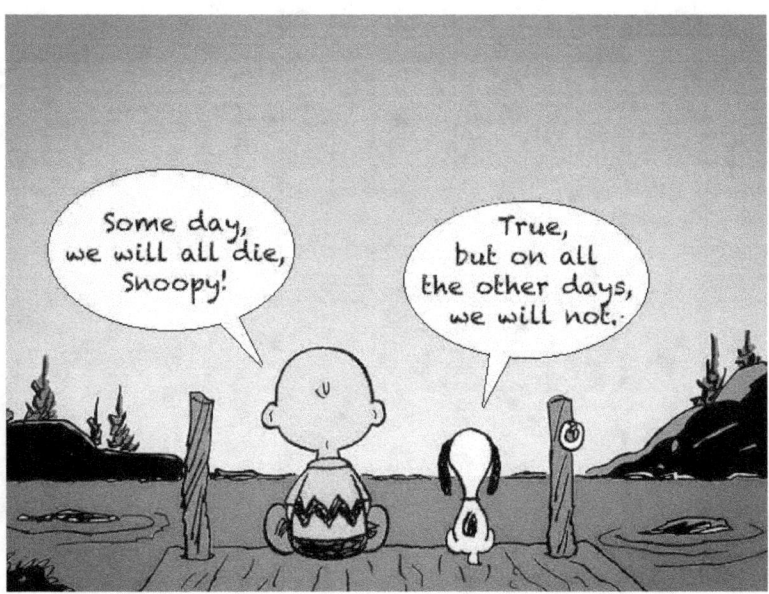

Thanks to Charles M. Schultz for Use of Snoopy & Charlie Brown